Here for good health.

About the Author

Originally from Mexico, Itzel has a long history in exercise and movement; she has been a Fitness Instructor and Personal Trainer since 2011, Leading groups and coaching individuals into getting great results through great posture, form and performance.

Itzel started her career as a Personal Trainer with the mantra: workouts should be fun, effective and easy to do, anytime and anywhere – and that has been the slogan of her career.

Founder of myBodyin.com and creator of myBodyin Shape, a metabolic conditioning series of linked exercises that combine high intensity workouts with strength training and a made-for-you-and-by-you easy to follow food menu that burns fat fast and slims the body down from all those troublesome areas. Her dedication, hard work and positivity make her a great and very popular trainer to work with and follow.

Fit & Slim for Life

Fit & Slim for Life

TABLE OF CONTENTS

Chapter Four

HOW TO FIRE UP YOUR METABOLISM:

THE METABOLIC CONDITIONING

I.   Fast Metabolism Fuel #1:

    EXERCISE SMART

II.   Fast Metabolism Fuel #2:

    EAT RIGHT

III.   Fast Metabolism Fuel #3:

    DE-STRESS

Chapter Five

TO BE FIT & SLIM FOR LIFE:

FIRE UP YOUR METABOLISM NOW!

Chapter Six

CHOOSING THE HEALTHY LIFESTYLE: The secrets of

staying Fit & Slim for life

Recipe Book

'Each morning, we are
born again.
What we do today is

what matters most'

- Buddha

Fit & Slim for Life

Introduction

If you have heard about metabolism, chances are it is in relation to weight loss. Metabolism is bigger than weight loss, though, as you will learn later on. It is about a healthier, better you.

If you want to fire up your metabolism and do not have any idea how to do it, you have come to the right place. If you have tried to speed up your metabolism before but do not see visible results, you have also come to the right place.

This book will walk you through the basics of metabolism and all that you need to do to speed up your metabolism.

Enjoy the trip! And don't forget to take the lessons home with you.

Chapter One

YOUR METABOLISM

MASERTERING THE BASICS

Metabolism Defined

Metabolism, in its most basic sense, is the body's conversion of the calories from the food you eat into energy. It is a series of chemical reactions that give your body the energy to do what it needs to do to keep functioning – and consequently, for you to keep living. Without metabolism, you would not be able to move or think. Metabolism provides energy for your body and your individual organs to work smoothly [Bosello 01,02].

To better understand the importance of metabolism, consider this: if your heart stops beating, you die.

Likewise, if your metabolism stops, you die – because without metabolism, you will not have the energy even to breathe, or for your heart to beat!

How Metabolism Works

First, let us start with the act of eating. As you chew and swallow your food, it goes down to your digestive tract. Digestive enzymes then break down your food – carbohydrates to glucose, fats into fatty acids, and protein into amino acids. After the nutrients are effectively broken down, they are absorbed by the bloodstream and are carried over to the cells.

Other enzymes plus hormones then work to either convert these nutrients into cells or building blocks for tissues or release them as an energy supply for the body's immediate use [Bosello 01,02].

The Metabolic Process

There are two basic metabolic processes – one is constructive, and is responsible for building and storing energy for the body. The other is destructive, though in a positive sense, as it breaks down nutrient molecules to release energy.

The constructive metabolic process is called anabolism, while the destructive process is called catabolism.

Anabolism promotes the growth of new cells, the maintenance and repair of tissues, and the storage of energy – usually through body fat – for future use. Small nutrient molecules are converted into larger molecules of protein, carbohydrates and fat.

Catabolism, meanwhile, is responsible for immediately providing the body energy to use. Instead of building up, it breaks down the nutrient molecules to release energy. These two processes do not occur simultaneously but are balanced by the body. Catabolism, in particular – though some attribute this to overall metabolism – has three components:

Fit & Slim for Life

1. **Basal metabolism.** Sometimes called resting metabolism, this is the metabolism component responsible for keeping you alive by ensuring normal body functions. Even if you were bedridden the whole day, basal metabolism is still at work, every time you breathe, digest, think or move you basal metabolism is at work, even when you are sleeping. People who want to lose weight usually aim for a higher basal metabolic rate (BMR).

Basal metabolism is metabolism's main component, as up to 65 percent of the calories from the food you eat are used for this. [F&NB 03]

2. **Physical movement.** This can range from a simple moving of your fingers to strenuous exercise.

Usually 25 percent of the calories you consume go here. [F&NB 03]

3. **Thermic effect of food.** This indicates the digestion and processing of the food you take in. Normally, 10 percent of   the calories of the food you eat are burned through this.

Fit & Slim for Life

Thus, taking all this into account, here is our metabolism formula:

Calories metabolized in 24 hours from the food you eat = Calories Expended From Basal Metabolism (60-70%) + Calories Expended By Physical Movement (25%) + Calories Expended Digesting Food (10%) [F&NB 03]

What Affects Metabolism?

Your metabolic rate, or how fast or slow your metabolism works, is influenced by a number of factors:

1. **Genetics.** Yes, metabolic rate is also inherited. Sometimes this makes an entire world of difference between a person who can eat almost everything and not gain an ounce and a person who easily balloons after indulging just once.

2. **Age.** The younger you are the faster your metabolism is. This is because growing and developing involves great amount of energy, up to the age of 21 you bones and muscles still growing and developing, using a great deal of energy and calories. Resistance training, more than aerobic training, has

been proven to maintain RMR levels by protecting and increasing muscle and bone structures as we age.

3. **Gender.** Men have a faster metabolic rate – usually 10-15 percent faster – than women because their bodies have a larger muscle mass. Muscle plays a key role in fast metabolism, as will be discussed in the chapter on how to Exercise Smart.

4. **Amount of lean body mass.** As already mentioned above, more muscle = faster metabolism.

5. **Diet.** Some foods will help you, some will only harm you. While timing is not everything, when you eat also greatly affects your metabolism. The difference is discussed in the chapter on how to Eat Right.

6. **Stress level.** Stress is inversely proportional to metabolism. The more stress you are subjected to, the lower your metabolism. You will better understand this when we move on to the chapter about how to De-stress.

7. **Hormones.** Specific hormones metabolize specific nutrients. How well the hormones work, then, directly affects

metabolism. To a certain extent, diet and stress levels affect the hormones involved in metabolism, as you will find out later. Hormonal disorders or imbalances can affect metabolism as well.

Looking at all these factors that influence metabolism, you now probably have a general idea of what you need to do to increase your metabolism – accept the things you cannot change, and work on those that you can!

But before we get into the detailed program for metabolic conditioning, first, know what's in it for you! And find out the kind of resolve you need to achieve the level of metabolism you want.

Does metabolic rate decline with age?

It's generally accepted that metabolic rate declines significantly as we age. Age related metabolic decline studies had shown, on average, that sedentary populations experience a 2 to 4% decline in resting metabolic rate (RMR) with each passing decade after the age of 25. However, this supposedly inevitable metabolic decline may be more lifestyle-related than age-related.

Researchers at the University of Colorado found that, amongst sedentary women, postmenopausal women between 50 and 72 years of age had significantly lower RMR than premenopausal women, providing evidence for age-related metabolic decline. However, the researchers found that RMR was not significantly different between premenopausal women and postmenopausal women who regularly performed endurance exercise. In fact, older women who regularly performed endurance exercise showed a higher RMR than some younger sedentary women. The conclusion of the study is 'Age-related decline in RMR in sedentary women is not observed in women who regularly perform endurance exercise. The elevated level of RMR observed in middle-aged and older exercising women may play a role in their lower levels of body weight and fatness compared to those in sedentary women'. [26]

In a follow-up study researchers compared a group of men age 19 to 36 years old and older, age 52 to 75 years old. They found that RMR was not significantly lower in older men who maintain exercise volume and energy intake at a level similar to that of young physically active men.

The researchers concluded that the decline on metabolic functions is not related to age, but to two controllable lifestyle factors: reduction in exercise volume (moving less) and reduction in energy intake (eating less). [27]

Chapter Two

WHY YOU SHOULD FIRE UP YOUR METABOLISM

It's not all about weight loss, though discussions on metabolism seem to focus almost exclusively on this concept. In fact, even if you feel that your weight is perfectly fine, you have a lot to gain by increasing your metabolism. Following a list of the benefits you stand to gain by applying the advice in this book:

1. **Lose weight**. Let's start with the most obvious benefit. By increasing your metabolism, particularly your BMR, you will burn more calories just by doing the activities you usually do. Even while you lie in bed and stare at the ceiling or even while you are sleeping, your body is working to burn the calories you consume. With an increase in metabolism, you can actually shed one or two pounds a week [MIA0 4,05]. Best of all, the results are long-term, unlike a quick-fix diet! Now, isn't that more satisfying – and easier – than going on a fad diet?

2. Eat more without worrying about it. Since you burn calories faster now, you can eat more without feeling guilty [MIA0 4,05]. This does not mean overindulging or snacking on junk food, though. But in general, you can be less concerned about the quantity of food you eat.

3. Feel more energized. People with faster metabolism report having more energy. With a faster metabolism, your body is performing efficiently to release the energy you need to get going.

4. Look better. The skin of people with a fast metabolism is brighter and more radiant. Their faces are pinkish, more alive with color. With a faster metabolism, you will not only feel good but also look good!

5. Be healthier overall. Your body functions more efficiently with a faster metabolism. Digestion, absorption of nutrients and blood circulation are improved. Hormonal balance.

In summary, a faster metabolism to make you look and feel wonderful!

Chapter Three

THE RIGHT MINDSET

FOR INCREASING YOUR METABOLISM

You are probably wondering what all this has to do with mindset. Why not go directly to the advice for increasing your metabolism?

The reason is that you need to be prepared for what lies ahead. Boosting your metabolism is a serious business. It is not like a quick-fix diet where you need only exert effort for a few weeks – and for some diets, even for a few days.

Boosting your metabolism is about changing your lifestyle and habits. Though you may choose to start with small changes, you will still be changing the way of life you have become used to – and it may feel uncomfortable at first. Boosting your metabolism requires discipline and consistency in your actions. And since you are expecting long-term results, you are likewise expected to make a long-term investment.

From here on, please look at the advice I will be presenting as an entire package or program. You cannot do only some of them and still get the same results. The tips here follow the gestalt principle – the whole is greater than the sum of the parts. Trust that the components of the program all work harmoniously to deliver your desired result.

So now I want you to close your eyes and imagine yourself – really imagine! – what you will be like after this program has started to take effect on you. How will you look? How will you feel?

Then, do the same process for your expectations after three months, then six months – or even a year, if you can. Note the differences you see and feel.

It's a good idea to write down your expected outcome. This will help you get through the program, especially when you are having a difficult time sticking to the changes you previously committed to.

Congratulations! You have just begun with the end in your mind. This will greatly help you along the way to your goal of firing up your metabolism.

You can always contact me if you need help or advise or if you are not sure how to do what or when to eat what, so ping me and email to itzel@mybodyin.com if you need help or visit my website www.mybodyin.com for tips.

Fit & Slim for Life

Chapter Four

HOW TO FIRE UP YOUR METABOLISM

As I mentioned, you will need to apply *all* the components in order to boost your metabolism and keep it fire up all the time, whatever you are doing, even if all you are doing is sitting on the sofa watching a movie.

First, we will talk about exercise, as an Exercise Professional this is what I do, focus on movement and exercise. But please be aware that in a weight loss program, exercise is always second to diet, you can't outrun a bad diet. Simply put, relying only on exercise to lose weight is not only hard and nearly impossible, but it will also take you a very long time, however exercise is crucial to achieve a lean and toned body and to look great. Exercise done right can greatly contribute to increasing your BMR [JAP 06]. Here, you will learn how to exercise smart, and not always hard, as some fitness programs might advise.

We will be talking about the importance of building muscle mass and applying the right intensity to exercise.

The second section is about eating right. Only second on this book's order, but remember, this is perhaps the most crucial element in the program– not about eating less, as some weight loss programs would advise – but eating smart. You will learn that the results you get will not only come from the food you eat, but *how* and *when* you eat as well.

The last section is about coping with stress. Some might see little importance in this section. Know, however, that stress is a real and strong impediment to boosting your metabolism. Bear this in mind as you read through this section.

Take time to absorb each piece of advice. You can start applying the advice here little by little, but with the intention of putting it all together once your body has adjusted.

Fast Metabolism Fuel #1:

EXERCISE SMART

Notice that I mentioned *smart,* not *hard.* Though some exercises here may be high-intensity and may indeed be hard for you, you need not work as long and as hard as you may think. The goal here is to fire up your metabolism with an exercise program that takes the shortest time[EA 07] and the least effort possible without sacrificing results, not at any point I am trying to hurt you, damage your joints or make you suffer. So learn to distinguish between sore muscle after a workout and the pain of an injury and stay safe, be smart.

I use a lot the sentence 'burn fat' for the purpose of this book and for you to understand what I mean. But I know that body fat doesn't burn, it metabolises [MIA 08]. I also know that long cardio workouts and non-challenging movements in fitness classes are fun, make you seat and get you tired, but do not get your body into metabolic conditioning.

To obtain Metabolic Conditioning, your workout must take your through the H's & B's [UNM0 9]. What I mean, is that an

Fit & Slim for Life

exercise qualifies as metabolically challenging if it is Heavy or challenging, creates Heat enough to make you sweat, makes you Breathless and you can feel the Burn during and after.

The two elements in this exercise program are strength and resistance training for building lean muscle mass and interval training for speeding up the metabolic process in general.

Strength and resistance training

The exercises under this training program are designed to literally build strength and resistance, as the name suggests. Tension is applied on the muscles to achieve this. The end result is increased muscle mass in your body.

Building muscle is important as more muscle in your body means more calories burned. Fitness trainer and consultant Robert Reames [RRT 10, 11 ,15]gives a perfect analogy by calling muscles fireplaces in the body that burn fuel – meaning calories. So the more fireplaces, the more fuel burned. For every pound of muscle added to your body, 40-50 calories more are burned per day [RRT 10, 11 ,15] .

Women need not worry about gaining large, unsightly muscles – your bodies are different from men. Your muscles will only add definition to your shape and in fact, make you look sexier. The combination of hormones in our bodies stop us from developing big muscles[RRT 10, 11 ,15] , so if you want to try bodybuilding, look for an specialist in the matter as this program will not increase your musculature to that degree.

While building muscles are usually associated with weight training, this is not always the case. There are in fact several exercises that do not require weights at all. If you are on a tight budget, you can in fact do exercises with no weights at all. For best results, though, do a combination of strength exercises with equipment and without equipment is recommended.

For clear differentiation, let us discuss weight lifting exercises first.

Weight lifting is a convenient muscle-building exercise as it applies tension to your muscles through an external source, the weights.

You can also easily measure your progress as the number of pounds or grams is indicated on each weight. As your body adjusts and strengthens, you can add more weights or replace your current weights with heavier ones.

To determine how many grams or pounds your weights should have, try them out first. The best weights for you are those that put tension in your muscles but do not make you feel fatigued. If you need help finding out how much weight you should lift, send me a message to itzel@mybodyin.com

The best exercises for achieving faster results for boosting metabolism are those that work several muscles in your body together. It's not a problem if you want to focus on a particular muscle, though, for example, if you want to tone or sculpt a specific body part.

There are many weight-lifting exercises you can choose from to include in your routine, but here are some basic examples:

1. **Bench press** – This is a multi-joint exercise, working the major muscles of the shoulders, chest and triceps. To do this,

lie on a bench and hold the weight over your chest with your elbows bent at 90 degrees. "Press" the weight up until your arms straighten, then lower it slowly back to your starting position.

2. **Chest fly** – This works the chest, with an emphasis on outer muscles. Lie on a bench with your weights held overhead, palms facing inward. Lower the weights to your sides up to shoulder level, with your elbows slightly bent. Slowly bring the weights up, back to starting position.

3. **Bicep curl** – This is one of the most basic weight lifting exercises. This puts effort on the biceps, as the name suggests. To do this, hold the weights with your palms facing out. Bend your elbows to bring the weights to your shoulders without touching them. Slowly lower the weights down, but do not straighten the arm out totally to keep a level of tension.

4. **Concentration curl** – This also works the biceps. Kneel on one leg using the leg opposite the hand you are working with. Hold one weight with your working hand and put the other hand on your waist. Place the back of the upper arm of your

working hand on the inner thigh of the other leg. You can lean into that leg to raise your elbow a little. Raise the weight to the front of your shoulder and then slowly lower the arm until almost straight.

5. **Overhead press** – This works the shoulder muscles. Stand or sit straight and hold your weights with your elbows bent and your hands in front of your eyes. Bring the weights over your head while keeping your back straight. Slowly bring the weights down to starting position.

Strength exercises without weights

Can be combined with weight lifting exercises for your routine.

Here are some examples:

1. **Squat** – A squat is a multi-joint exercise working the hamstrings, quadriceps, gluteals, and the lower back. In fact, this is one of the most effective strength exercises without weights. From a standing position, slowly lower your body until your knees bend at a 90-degree angle. Keep your feet flat on

the floor while doing this. Return to a standing position slowly as well.

2. Push-up – This is also a very typical but effective strength and resistance exercise. While the basic one works well, adding complexity can work more muscles. For example, you can do push-ups with you feet on an unstable surface, like a ball. Or hands in two balls, feet on the floor. Or one hand on one ball and change the ball to the other hand after every push-up. These challenge abs, chest and triceps.

3. Plank – Yes, the basic plank is a strength exercise, and done properly, it fires up all major muscles in the core. I am not a fan of crunches as an abs exercise, they put strain on the vertebrae of the neck, promote bad posture as to you are mainly training to round shoulders and done properly they are far too much hard work for just a couple of muscles properly involved in the workout. You are welcome to do crunches, but I will recommend better to try all forms of planks, leg extensions, weighted bridges and wood choppers for a better abdominal workout. For variety in exercises and for working different sets of muscles, you can also try working out with different equipment like exercise balls.

In planning your routine for strength exercises, refer to the body's muscle groups below and determine which you want to work on. Remember, though, that multi-joint exercises are still best to achieve faster metabolism [NCBI1 12,13].

1. **Biceps** – These are found at the front of your upper arm.

2. **Triceps** – These are at the back of your upper arm.

3. **Deltoids** – These are the caps of your shoulders.

4. **The Pectoralis major** – This is the large, fan-shaped muscle on the front of your upper chest.

5. **Rhomboids** – These are muscles in the middle of your upper back and located between the shoulder blades.

6. **Trapezius** – This is on your upper back, sometimes called 'traps.' The upper trapezius, in particular, runs from the back of your neck to your shoulder.

Fit & Slim for Life

7. **Latisimus dorsi** – These are large muscles that go down the middle of your back. When exercised well, they give your back an attractive V shape, giving the illusion of a smaller waist.

8. **Lower back** – This comprises the erector spine muscles that enable back extension. This also helps in maintaining good posture.

9. **Abdominals** – Of course! This is where the belly fat usually goes, the flab you want to banish forever. The abdominals are composed of the external obliques, which trace paths down the sides and the front of the abdomen, and the rectus abdominus, a flat muscle running across the abdomen.

10. **Gluteals** – Also called "glutes" the main muscle here is the gluteus maximus, the muscle on your buttocks.

11. **Quadriceps** – These muscles go up the front of your thigh.

12. **Hamstrings** – These are on the back of your thighs.

13.   Hip abductors and adductors – These are located at your inner and outer thigh. Abductors are on the outside, moving the leg away from your body. On the other hand, adductors are on the inside, pulling the leg to the center of your body.

14.   Calf – The calf muscles are on the back of the lower leg. The two calf muscles are the gastrocnemius and the soleus. The former gives the calf a stable, round shape while the soleus is a flat muscle below the gastrocnemius.

After choosing your exercises, you must think about the level of intensity and the duration of your exercises.

The number of repetitions and sets actually depends on your level of tolerance – fatigue is a sign that you have achieve intensity, but also a sign that you have overtaxed yourself, you must make sure you know the difference.

Let yourself feel the "burn" in your muscles or the soreness but do not push yourself more than you can go. In general, though, the American College of Sports Medicine recommends three sets or more of strength exercises with six to eight repetitions for each set for building muscle [ACS 14,17]. If you are a beginner, though, it may take time before you reach this level. Not more than a 45-second rest should be taken between sets for best results in increasing metabolism.

Your exercise routine can last for only 30 minutes or less and still achieve optimum results.

At this point, I want to emphasize that strength and resistance exercises are the best *and* healthiest way to build muscles. Do not ever look for shortcuts, like performance-enhancing drugs or steroids with growth hormones.

While they may help increase your muscle mass, they can have side effects such as heart attacks, liver damage, and even premature death. It is best for you to stick to the healthy and proven methods in building muscles.

The benefits of strength exercises are also numerous and not merely confined to boosting metabolism. They lower blood pressure, improve balance and flexibility, increase your stamina for other activities, and reduce your risk of injury – as these are strength exercises, they in fact strengthen your muscles and bones!

Metabolic Chain Workout

A metabolic chain workout is long chain of exercises performed back-to-back in one seamless compact movement that increases your body's metabolic demand, increasing fat burn during the time you exercise and long after you finish in the gym, creating the very beneficial after-burn we have talk about.

But there is one important element that allows targeted muscle growth and progressive resistance. Each exercise in the chain has a single repetition added in each round and deducted at the end of the series: with dumbbells in hands do the following sequences of exercises.

Shoulder upright row, followed by Shoulder over head push, followed by forward row elbows lead to back, followed by side rise, followed by a squat, followed by lunge right and left, followed by ½ burpee and a push-up, complete the burpee and stand tall.

Fit & Slim for Life

Now, repeat this entire sequence of movements except this time do two of each movement including two push-ups. On the third round, do three moves. On the fourth round, do 4 of each move and so on and so forth until you reach 6 of each move. Now, reverse the pyramid start from doing 6 moves of each and slowly work your way back down the compact chain pyramid until you do 1 move of each. Then repeat again and again working up the chain to 6 moves and then down to 1. Go up and down the pyramid as many times as you can with good form.

Continue like this for 15 minutes resting whenever it is required and continuing exactly where you left off. At the end of 15 minutes stop wherever you are. It is best to record the total number of push-ups you completed.

This gives you a baseline measure to attempt to beat next time.

Fit & Slim for Life

Interval training

These exercises are about "intervals", or "on – off sets" referring to high-intensity exercise and rest. In this training, you do a cardiovascular exercise at the highest intensity you can manage, then shift to a moderate/low intensity for rest, do high intensity again, then moderate/low, and so on. Reames calls this "metabolic burst" training [RRT 10, 11 ,15], as the sudden burst you do in the high-intensity exercise also results in a burst of calorie-burning. Because of the sudden "burst" you give to your body, it also suddenly releases energy. The rest period, meanwhile, is essential for the body to get rid of the waste products in the muscles you are using in the exercise. It is important to keep a moderate intensity of exercise and not go into total rest.

This is to ensure that the release of energy is continuous.

Interval training can be done for almost any type of cardiovascular exercise – running, biking, swimming, and more. For running, the rest period can be brisk walking; for biking and swimming, the activity can be done at a slower but moderate pace. The high-intensity and moderate-intensity exercise can also be slightly different. For example, the high-intensity exercise may be briskly walking up the stairs while the low-intensity exercise may be brisk walking on a flat surface.

Each interval should last between one to four minutes. The rest period can be shorter or longer than your high-intensity exercise, depending on your condition. Doing your interval training routine for a total of 20 minutes already achieves optimal results.

Just ensure that your moderate-intensity exercise really still *has* intensity while allowing your body to rest for the next burst of high-intensity exercise. Perform your personal best for the high-intensity exercise – being almost out of breath is a good sign.

A more accurate way of determining the highest level of intensity you can manage is by calculating your maximum heart rate. To get your maximum heart rate, simply subtract

Fit & Slim for Life

your age from 220 [ACC 16]. During exercise, a heart rate monitor will come in handy although this is optional. To monitor your heart rate manually, find your pulse in your wrist then count the number of beats within six seconds. Put the number zero at the end of that. If you counted 16 beats, your pulse rate is 160 beats per minute. Your pulse rate after high-intensity exercise should be 75-85 percent of your maximum heart rate. Your pulse rate during moderate-intensity exercise should always be greater than your resting heart rate or your normal heart rate when you are not doing any exercise. Again, to get your resting heart rate, get your pulse rate while you are not doing exercise.

For those who want to boost metabolism primarily to lose weight, here's the good news: after a few weeks of interval training, expect even your normal exercise with moderate intensity to burn more fat than usual.

A study by exercise scientist Jason Talanian supports this claim[NCB 18]. After seven interval workouts distributed over two weeks, subjects increased their fat burning by 36 percent through normal cycling exercises only.

Also, after interval training comes the excess post-exercise oxygen consumption (EPOC), better known as the "metabolic after-burn" [JOA 19] this means that your body continues burning calories for up to *46 hours* after your workout. Interval training sure beats normal cardiovascular training. Also, normal cardiovascular exercise usually takes longer as the objective is endurance. Contrast this with interval training which only requires 20 to 30 minutes or even less and which delivers significant results in just a few weeks.

Putting it all together

While you will be choosing your specific exercises for the strength and resistance training and interval training, I will be recommending an exercise schedule and giving you tips for your best application of the exercises.

Below would be the best weekly schedule for your workout:

Day 1: Strength and resistance exercises

Day 2: Interval training exercises

Day 3: Strength and resistance exercises / or Metabolic chain workout

Day 4: Interval training exercises / or Rest

Day 5: Metabolic chain workout / or Strength and resistance exercises

Day 6: Interval training exercises

Day 7: Rest

As you can see, strength exercises and interval training are done on alternate days. This is to facilitate recovery of the muscles you use. As your training progresses and you grow fitter and stronger, increase the times a week you put exercises together in a Metabolic Chain Workout from once a week up to 3 times a week, do not ever over do the metabolic chains workout and always allow your body to recover.

Do not ever, ever do your strength exercise workout right after your interval training workout – this will slow down the process of muscle building.

One day or two without exercise during the week is also crucial for your body to make a full recovery. Taking two days rest doesn't mean you are weak, but that you are getting stronger as the intensity rises also should increase your rest periods.

Again, I would like to emphasize that you should never push your body to pain or extreme fatigue.

Doing so would trigger a stress response in your body, which may have serious effects on your metabolism.

The link between stress and metabolism will be discussed in a later section.

Also, make sure that you breathe normally throughout the exercises so that your body is not stressed.

Always perform warm-up exercises before your routine and cool-down exercises after. For a warm-up, a cardio of moderate intensity and arm circling would be a good example. For a cool-down, a total body stretch will relax your muscles. Breathing exercises will also help in relaxing.

You can apply variety to your exercise routines to work different muscles and for your own enjoyment, especially if you get bored with the same exercise routines.

Fit & Slim Checkpoint:

Before we proceed

Here are some more things to think about as you plan your exercise program to fire up your metabolism:

1. **Age does not matter.** Yes, whether you are 20 or 60, you can trust that the exercise program we discussed will work for you. For older people, your interval training may not be as intense at first, but after some time, you just might be surprised how far your body can go. Looking at strength and resistance training in particular: here's something for older people to consider: a scientific study conducted at Tufts university shows that age is not an obstacle to building muscle. In their study, 87- to 96-year-old women who underwent an 8-week strength training program tripled their strength and increased their muscle by ten percent [JOA 20].

2. **Other exercise is good, but...** I recommend you not to overdo it and to apply the exercise program discussed here. While it is true that any physical activity burns calories, it only has a one-time effect. The exercises here, however, are guaranteed to have a long-term effect. Also, endurance training is good, but you will get more and faster results from interval training. You can try new exercises, and specially to create your own Metabolic Chain Workouts, you can get creative and link together all kind of exercises, but be careful

and overall, be SMART. Don't overdo it and don't ever overwork one part of your body as this only will slow you down, make you susceptible to injury and may even be more harmful that helpful to your training progress.

3. More exercise does not mean faster metabolism.

Logically, more exercise means more calories burned. But as your goal here is a long-term increase in your metabolism, you should not be obsessed by how much you exercise but on the quality of your exercise. Again, this deserves repetition – do not push yourself beyond your limits as it will drive your body into a stress reaction. Stress has a serious effect on metabolism.

So now you know the best exercise program to fire up your metabolism. But don't stop reading just yet – exercise is only one part of your journey to a faster metabolism.

Fast Metabolism Fuel #2:

EAT RIGHT, BE SMART

You wouldn't put into a Ferrari 458 Spider a mixture of low quality fuel, sugar and cheap fats, would you? You will put the best fuel for this amazing machine to give you its best performance.

Food is your main fuel for energy – it gives your body the calories it processes to burn or to store energy. The right food, the right amount the right quality, and the right time in eating will give you the best results possible for your metabolism.

For all those who are trying to lose weight, you need to know that eating to boost metabolism is radically different from traditional weight loss diets. In traditional diets, calories, fat or carbohydrates are your enemy and you have to monitor your calorie intake, but the opposite is true for the fast metabolism diet. Calories are now your friends – the good calories, at least.

Remember when we talked about exercise? The more muscles you build, the more calories you burn. And after you've done interval training for a while, your body also burns more calories. So to keep up with the calorie burning, you actually have to eat more. You will understand this better later.

Nutrients to Befriend

Carbohydrates are one of the most essential nutrients for firing up your metabolism. They are the most basic fuel for the energy you consume for physical activities. If you exercise regularly, carbohydrates are necessary. But if you are building muscle, carbohydrates are *crucial.* As you progress in your muscle building and interval training, you need to increase your carbohydrate intake.

As your body burns more energy, it will need more energy from carbohydrates. If the carbohydrates you consume are not enough, your body will turn to your muscle mass and get its energy there. Yes, your hard-worked muscles will be wasted if you do not consume enough carbohydrates.

More than 50 percent of your calorie requirements should come from carbohydrates, in the form of vegetables, roots, fruits, pulses and unprocessed grains.

There are two types of carbohydrates – simple and complex. Simple carbohydrates are easier to digest and absorb compared with complex carbohydrates. If we are to consider the thermic effect of food which also contributes to faster metabolism, complex carbohydrates are the way to go.

And usually, complex carbohydrates are the healthy types of food while the simple carbohydrates are usually the processed foods loaded with preservatives and artificial sweeteners.

For complex carbohydrates you have a wider range of options.

Below few examples.

Complex Carbohydrates:

Grains and Cereals: Oatmeal, whole wheat bread, whole wheat pasta, brown rice, bran corn, etc

Fit & Slim for Life

<u>Root Crops:</u> Potato, sweet potato, yam, manioc, etc.

<u>Vegetables:</u> Broccoli, cauliflower, cabbage, eggplant, cucumber, salads, green leafy vegetables, all peppers, tomatoes, squash, asparagus, onions, garlic, etc.

Yes, carbohydrates are not all grains and root crops. We have fibrous, high in water content carbohydrates as well – the vegetables. The fiber, though not absorbed by the digestive system, helps in the thermic effect. Fiber also cleanses the body and thus ensures its smooth functioning, including the enzymes and hormones for metabolism.

Protein is another essential nutrient in the diet for faster metabolism. Protein is processed by the body into amino acids, the building block for cells – and consequently, muscles. And, like complex carbohydrates, protein also has a thermic effect as it takes a long time for the body to break it down.

Proteins are known as the building blocks of life: they promote cell growth and repair.

They also take longer to digest than carbohydrates, helping you feel fuller for longer and on fewer calories, a plus for anyone trying to lose weight.

Below are some healthy, excellent sources of protein:

1. **Chicken** – Go for the breast, as it has the highest amount of protein. Drumsticks are also good, though not so high in protein. Just remove the skin to get rid of saturated fat and cholesterol.

2. **Fish** – This is good protein without the bad, unlike red meat. Aside from having high protein content, it is also good for the heart, particularly cold-water fish like salmon and tuna.

3. **Eggs** – Very rich in protein and affordable too. Eggs contain all the essential amino acids for growth. Contrary to what some may think, the high protein content comes mostly from the egg white and not the egg yolk.

4. **Red lean meat** – High in Iron, not only so important for ladies that work out, but for all, men and women physically active. It forms complexes bindings with

molecular oxygen in hemoglobin and myoglobin; these two compounds are essential in oxygen and proteins transport in the body. Iron is also the metal at the active site of many important enzymes dealing with cellular respiration and oxidation reduction at cellular level, it is the ultimate antioxidant.

5. **Whey** – Though not a natural whole food, whey is very high in protein and is also healthy. It is a staple among body builders. Whey is sold as protein powder.

6. **Vegetarian proteins** – Evidence suggest that vegetarians have lower rates of coronary heart disease obesity, hypertension, type 2 diabetes and osteoporosis[JOA 21]. Vegetarian proteins like pulses, quinoa, nuts and green-leaf vegetables are generally low in saturated fat, cholesterol and can be adequate for a healthy living as long as they are varied and provide all nutrients needed.

Fats are also essential for fast metabolism. Now, this may raise a few eyebrows, especially among those who have tried conventional weight loss diets. This is where the fast metabolism diet, again, sets itself apart. While too much fat – especially unhealthy fat – is bad, a small amount of healthy fats helps hormones responsible for metabolism to continue performing well. Diets low in fat lead to poor hormone production, and thus, slower metabolism.

When adding fats to your diet remember to keep the naturally sourced and avoid any man made type of fat, like the one find in diet and low-fat products. Healthy sources of fat are olive oil, avocados, sunflower seeds, coconut oil, oily fish, and nuts.

As with fats, **calcium** helps release hormones that boost metabolism. Milk, of course, is the best source of calcium. Yogurt is also high in calcium and has other health benefits as well.

"Nutrients" to Avoid

As a piece of advice for good health and long life, avoid empty calories like the plague. These come from refined, highly processed foods – usually the simple, over-processed carbohydrates that are not natural whole foods. Why empty calories? They fill you up but give little or no nutrients. What's more, these foods usually contain a lot of sugar – and too much sugar seriously affects the metabolism.

Just to drive home the point, below are examples of foods with empty calories:

All sweats and candies, gums and jellies, chocolate, sweat bred, cakes, pastries, biscuits, packaged meals, takeaway meals, bread, flat bread, wraps, pastas, pizza, processed cured meats, margarine, light or diet products, fizzy, low calorie and flavored drinks, fruit juices, all colorants. As general rule, stay clear of all products made in a factory like salad cream, mayonnaise and other sauces.

I would recommend you to get use to reading the product labels, if you can't pronounce an ingredient, you better no eat it.

Too much caffeine is also not good for your metabolism. It triggers a stress response. So go easy on the coffee.

Other Recommended Foods (22)

1. **Spices** – Cayenne pepper and red hot pepper, in particular, contain capsaicin which is said to raise metabolism up to 25 percent for three hours. Cinnamon is great to help with keeping blood sugar balanced. Using herbs and spices instead of salt when you cook, will keep your heart healthy.

2. **Green Tea** – It's not all about antioxidants. Taken regularly, green tea can increase the thermic effect of food. Research from the University of Geneva shows that green tea speeds up fat oxidation in addition to boosting metabolism.

   Green tea also has less caffeine than coffee, whose caffeine level may greatly affect metabolism. For those who do not like the bitter taste, green tea extract is available in capsule form.

3. **Coconut Oil - cold-pressed**

While olive oil has always been and will continue to be a staple, highly nutritious and recommended for a healthy lifestyle, there's a new kid on the block that is getting all the attention, and for many good reasons. Coconut oil, which is actually 90% saturated fat, is the new superstar in the kitchen. But how something so high in saturated fat can be any good for us? Even more than just good for you, coconut oil may help you to lose weight.

Let me explain, cold-pressed vegetable oils are actually good for us; they are full of fatty essential acids, essential vitamins and omega oils, especially Omega-6, virgin olive oil being at the top to the list.

The trouble starts when we cook with the oil. Increasing the temperature of oil, as in cooking, frying or baking transforms the goodness of vegetable oil into hydrogenated and partially hydrogenated fats, these are essentially the bad guys and they are pretty bad for your health. So when you cook a nutritious meal with nutritious olive oil, is just as bad as cooking with fat substitutes and margarines, you are saturating the food with dangerous and highly toxic Trans fats. Not a good idea.

But coconut oil reacts different in the presence of heat. It has a very high resistance to temperature, which means that it will not mutate as you cook and your stir-fry will be just as healthy before and after cooking it, and you will get an all-natural food chockfull of health-building saturates fats.

According with Alexandra Bernardin from the Poliquin Group [BA 28], we should all increase our consumption of Coconut Oil because:

•   It's composed of medium chain triglycerides (MCTs), which your body can quickly and efficiently use for energy and may not be stored in the body as fat.

•   Coconut oil is high in lauric acid, which plays a critical role in immune system function.

•   It is high in antioxidants like capric acid and caprlic acid.

•   It is antiviral, antifungal, anti-parasite and anti-protozoa.

•   Populations that consume 30-60 percent of their daily caloric intake from coconuts are virtually free from cardiovascular disease and present lower cholesterol than those consuming other vegetable oils and fats, showing evidence that may have cardio protective attributes.

•   Unlike unsaturated vegetable oils like soybean and corn oil, coconut oil does not block or impair the secretion of thyroid hormone, helping to improve and maintain metabolic functions.

- Coconut oil is easily digested and may support healthy digestive function, as well as helping with zinc and magnesium absorption.

In addition, several studies have linked the consumption of cold-pressed coconut oil to smaller waist sizes. For example, researches at the Faculdade de Nutricao, Universidade Federal de Alagoas found that subjects who consumed two tablespoons of coconut oil per day for 12 weeks while following a reduced-calorie diet and including walking as daily exercise lost a significant amount of abdominal fat compared to the control group that followed the same diet and exercise program without coconut oil. In addition, the coconut oil group also experienced a significant decrease in their LDL:HDL cholesterol ration. The conclusion of this series of studies states, 'Supplementation with coconut oil does not cause dyslipidemia (elevation of plasma cholesterol, triglycerides or both) and seems to promote a reduction in abdominal obesity.'[ASS 29]

Water is life – and fuel – for metabolism

The old advice holds true for overall health as well as metabolism – drink at least eight glasses of water a day. Drink when you are thirsty and prefer fresh, clear unadulterated water than any flavored drink.

Dehydration affects metabolism through a drop in body temperature [BCOWL 23]. This drop triggers your body to store fat to help increase or maintain your body temperature.

Also, as you will be doing more exercises, you need water to keep your energy levels. If you sweat a lot, you should drink more water – even more than the eight glasses.

Water cleanses the body of toxins and thus enables body processes to proceed smoothly, including metabolism.

Timing is key in eating

Even though you are consuming the right foods, your results will be compromised if your timing is not perfect. Follow the advice below and you will get the best results.

1. **Eat several meals a day, every two and a half hours to three hours.** To really maximize the thermic effect of food, you need to eat more than the usual three meals. Eating every three hours will allow the thermic effect to last you throughout the day, as it takes between two and a half to three hours to digest food while protein broken down to amino acids stays for three hours in the bloodstream. For the exact number of meals, the magic number for men is six while it is five for women. Men require 600-900 more calories every day than women.

Do not go over your optimal number of meals, especially through late night snacking. When you are asleep, your body has a difficult time digesting. Also, the calories from your last meal are stored as fat.

Keeping the last meal light and easier to digest compared with the earlier meals is recommended.

2. **Always eat breakfast.** Your body has been in starvation mode during your sleep time. To get your metabolism up and running again, start the day right with a healthy, hearty

Fit & Slim for Life

breakfast. The later you eat your first meal for the day, the later your metabolism starts.

3. **Do not skip meals.** Under no circumstances should you skip meals, especially the three basic meals. If you have a busy schedule and have a hard time snacking, keep "emergency" foods within your reach, like whole wheat crackers and bananas. During particularly hectic days, just a few crackers or one banana would suffice as a snack to keep your metabolism running. A fresh fruit shake or a protein shake would also be enough.

4. **Take one snack or meal after your workout.** A meal or snack with protein and carbohydrates taken within one hour after your workout for the day helps in the recovery of your muscles and the building of new ones.

5. **Do not eat less than two and a half hours before bedtime.** Though metabolism still happens while sleeping, digestion will be difficult and your calories will most likely be stored as fat in your body.

Putting it all together

Fit & Slim for Life

The following advice is given in general terms, but please do remember, we are all different metabolically and different foods have different effects in different people, for example, you may be able to eat diary or not at all.

The majority of people will metabolise food and storage fat for the following groups. So let's start by following a simple rule, eat more of the green food category, eat none or very little of the red category. Eat from the yellow category with caution.

Green Food Group: eat unlimited, fill up your plate form this list

•   Protein and lean meat: chicken, turkey, wild fowl, game meats, fish, bison, lean ground beef, shellfish, lean cuts of pork, egg whites and high quality no sugar added protein powder.

•   Non-starch high-fiber veggies: kale, collards, Brussels sprouts, broccoli, all cabbage, cauliflower spinach, lettuce, salad greens, tomato, jicama, asparagus, green beans, runner beans, cucumber celery, peppers, carrots, radish, zucchini, squashes, pumpkin, leek, pok choi, etc.

- High-water, low-sugar fruits: all berries, apples, pears and all citrus fruit.

- Dairy substitutes: almond and rice milk with no added sugar

Yellow Food Group: **eat to tolerance**

o   Protein and fatty meat: lamb, fatty cuts of beef, fatty cuts of pork, sausages (80% meat), bacon, hams from cured meat yoke and whole eggs.

o   Vegetable fats: avocado, olives, olive oil, coconut oil, vegetable oils, nuts and seeds, not sugar added nuts butter.

o   Lower-fiber, high-sugar fruits: bananas, melons, cherries pineapple, mango, kiwi, exotic fruits like papaya, passion fruit and watermelon, all homemade juices and smoothies

o   Starchy low-fiber veggies and wet starches: all potatoes varieties corn and sweat corn, peas, sweet potatoes, rice, quinoa, oats, cuscus, bans and legumes.

○   Dairy: milk, yogurt, butter, cheese (full or half fat)

Reed Food Group: **eat rarely if ever, the nutritional content on this group is so low in quality and quantity that makes it 'better not to eat'**

▪   All refined products, if it has a 'list of ingredients' it has been processed. If any part of this list you cannot pronounce, leave it alone!

○   Dry starches: pasta, bread, crackers, chips, crisps, rice cakes, cereals, cereal bars

○   Junk food: cookies, sweats, jelly sweats, packed juices and shop bought smoothies, deep fried food and takeaways, baked goods, diet products, carbonated drinks, milks shakes, ice-creams, etc.

Sample meal plans

Below are two sample meal plans for a day. The key in each meal, particularly the main ones, is to combine protein and carbohydrates. Portions depend on your personal daily calorie requirements. Remember, though, that carbohydrates should have the biggest share in your diet – and these include hefty servings of vegetables! – followed by protein. Calcium is also essential. Fats are the least priority. You can include green tea with your meals – six cups throughout the day is best.

MEAL PLAN 1

6 AM - Meal 1

Oatmeal with banana slivers

Poached egg

9 AM - Meal 2

Protein Shake

1 PM - Meal 3

Skinless chicken breast drizzled with olive oil

 Brown rice

Steamed broccoli

4 PM - Meal 4

Green beans

Potatoes

Fit & Slim for Life

7 PM - Meal 5

Salmon fillet

Sweet potato

Cauliflower

MEAL PLAN 2

6 AM - Meal 1

Egg white pancakes (only one or two yolks can be added)

Choice of fruit/s – banana, blueberry and/or strawberries

9 AM - Meal 2

Yogurt

Choice of fruit

1 PM - Meal 3

Vegetable curry

Brown rice

4 PM - Meal 4

Fruit salad with greens and grilled chicken

(Note: dressing should ideally be vinaigrette, with olive oil)

Fit & Slim for Life

7 PM - Meal 5

Chili (made of turkey, kidney beans and salsa)

Steamed vegetables

These meal plans are here just to give you an idea. Create your own, but remember the principles. You can also change the times here, but remember not to eat too late at night.

Fit & Slim Checkpoint:

Below are just some warnings and some things to watch out for in eating and nutrition for faster metabolism:

1. **Some foods can only take you so far.** Spicy foods and green tea do have some effect in boosting metabolism, but only as an addition to a diet already rich in protein and carbohydrates. Relying on these alone for your diet for faster metabolism is not enough, but they are a great idea on to complement you natural healthy diet.

2. **Some foods won't take you there at all.** Some foods like celery (full or juiced), maple syrup and grapefruit especially are

popular among dieters as its high acidity, fiber or magic ingredient is perceived to burn fats. However, there is no scientific proof for any of this.

Same thing with all those fab diets based on one food only. So be carefully on taking one food only diets.

3. **No supplement will boost your metabolism.** To those who are taking supplements to boost your metabolism, you may just be wasting your money. Again, there is no scientifically proven link between supplements and faster metabolism.

4. **Diet pills are a no-no.** For those who want to lose weight, some diet pills may burn some fat and control your appetite. However, they do NOT boost metabolism. Also, the downside of diet pills is that once you get used to a certain dose, you need to take more to get the same effect as before. A few of those diet pills out there may indeed boost metabolism, but can have serious side effects. Read the box or container carefully. Better yet, consult your doctor. Looking at the adverse effects diet pills can have, wouldn't you prefer to

boost your metabolism the natural way? You will look and feel better.

3. **Organic is best.** If you think about all the food that is produced and the speed it needs to be produced to feed us all, then you'll realise that an immense amount of chemicals go in the food we consume. Chemicals that are not good for your body or your metabolism. So choose a respectable, sustainable source to get the meat, fish and vegetables you consume. Your body and the planet will be better for it.

No time to think about your diet? If you only take one piece of advice from this section, make sure it is this:

EAT FOOD

Fresh fruit, vegetables, wholegrain, pulses and seeds

Organic / from a respectable source

Omegas – feed your brain – fish, green veggies, nuts and seeds

Drink Water

AVOID CRAP

Carbonated drinks / Caffeine in excess

Refined sugars and white food – white bread, flour, sugar, pasta

Artificial sweeteners / Artificial Fats (hydrogenated or trans-fats)

Processed food – if it comes in a box or colorful package (including take away, supermarket ready to eat food)

We are now on the last leg of the program to fire up your metabolism. Keep reading!

Fast Metabolism Fuel #3:

DE-STRESS

You might be wondering what the purpose of this section is – isn't stress supposed to be a daily, ordinary part of life? But that is just the point. We now live in a fast-paced culture driven by urgency and deadlines. The more things you get done in less time, the better. Work, family and recreation have become a balancing act. Tension, worry, anxiety and fear are all too common. Emotional problems like failure in marriages, deaths of loved ones, or simply troubled relationships are accompanied with pressures from work.

Stress, especially prolonged exposure to stress, can seriously affect your metabolism, as well as your overall health and well-being.

The stress and metabolism link

There is a hormone in our body called cortisol [JBS 24], which aids in certain body functions. It aids regulation of blood pressure, release of insulin for blood sugar stability, increase of immunity, and proper metabolism of glucose. Small increases of cortisol can be beneficial, resulting in a quick, healthy jolt of energy and immunity, heightened memory, and a higher pain threshold. However, when too much cortisol is released or if it is released too often, it results in the following:

Blood sugar imbalances
Higher blood pressure
Decreased immunity
Lower cognitive performance
Decrease in bone density
Decrease in muscle tissue

Cortisol particularly stimulates amino acid release from your muscles to be converted to glucose that will serve as an energy source for your body to cope with stress. Yes, your hard-earned muscles are at the mercy of cortisol if you don't control its levels in your body.

The release of cortisol is mainly triggered by stress, whether physical or emotional in nature. Remember what we talked about for your exercise routine? Do not overtax yourself as it triggers the body's stress response.

Stress is also harmful to the body as it leads to the production of more acid than the body needs. Our bodies usually have an 80 percent alkaline and 20 percent acid balance. More acid in the body will upset that balance. Too much acid decreases your immunity and makes you more vulnerable to illness. Too much acid also affects body functions, including metabolism[JBS2].

You can effectively cope with stress and keep your cortisol levels healthy and stable, though. When your body goes into the stress response, it is important that you help it go into the relaxation response.

Less Stress = higher calorie burn

New research suggests the body burns fewer calories when we're under pressure or suffering from stress or stress related lack of sleep. The study in Biological Psychiatry followed a group of women from different ages and backgrounds for 10 days. The researchers asked the women to eat a high –fat meal followed by a 30 min leisure walk every day. The researchers then measured how much energy they used, as well as their blood sugar, insulin, fat and cortisol (the stress hormone) levels. They also monitored the women's stressful experiences. The results showed that those who experienced stressful events the day before used less energy after the meal, lower fat oxidation and higher insulin levels. In total, stressed women burned 104 fewer calories every day. Add that up over the course of a year and it would amount to an 11-pound weight gain! [27]

Ways to de-stress

There are many ways to de-stress, as there are many causes of stress. Pick the ones to your liking, try new things, and get creative: too long in front of the TV monitor is not really de-stressing.

1. **Aromatherapy** – This is particularly effective to let your stress during the day dissipate. Lavender and mint essential oils have excellent relaxing properties. A few drops mixed with water on your oil burner will suffice. You can also combine aromatherapy with meditation. As the aroma envelops you, feel it slowly sucking in your tiredness and worries. As the aroma leaves later on, imagine that your tiredness and worries are also going away with it.

You can also briefly relax with aromatherapy during work. Put a few drops on a piece of tissue paper and inhale.

2. **Massage** – This is also aptly called touch therapy. A massage is also beneficial as it loosens the muscles and joints that may have tensed up due to continuous stress. Back muscles are particularly susceptible to this. You can also

combine massage with aromatherapy – you can ask the masseur or masseuse to use essential oils for your massage. Peppermint is particularly excellent. Aside from its aroma, it has a cooling effect on the body when used as massage oil.

3. **Music therapy** – Put some gentle, relaxing music on your player, sit or lie in a comfortable position, close your eyes, and let the music wash over you. Imagine it washing away your worries, fears, and anxieties. A good alternative to soothing music is the sounds of nature, like ocean waves. Recordings of nature sounds are available in music stores. If you find you enjoy relaxing on the beach, then bring the beach home with you through a recording of ocean waves.

4. **Imagery** – Imagine that you are a kite slowly rising and floating through the air. You float in the bright blue sky in perfect balance and harmony with the wind. After some time, feel yourself slowly gliding downwards and then softly touching the ground.

The above imagery is particularly helpful not only for relaxing but for simulating a good response to stress – notice that the motion of the kite is in harmony with the wind, when the same wind can also make the kite spin out of control.

Another imagery technique is to imagine a beautiful scene from nature like a mountaintop, a secluded island, or a tropical rain-forest. Imagine yourself, from a first-person perspective, walking through the place and taking in all the beauty.

You can vary the place you visit every time you use this technique, or you can pick one and make it your sanctuary – the place you flee to during moments of stress.

Make it a long term practice:

1. Think positive! – Thoughts greatly influence your health and well-being. Your thoughts can actually manifest into reality, as maintained by philosophers, contemporary speakers and even scientists. So bad thoughts can manifest negatively, while positive thoughts manifest positively. So if you are going to think, you might as well think of pleasant things. If you have anxieties over something, like an upcoming presentation for work, imagine yourself – from the first-person perspective – giving an excellent, flawless presentation. Imagine the reactions of your audience. Feel the feelings as if you were there already. Images are more powerful than words, so apply the same principle to your thoughts.

2. **Let go of negative feelings.** Wallowing in negative feelings equals more acid in the body. No wonder tension and fear lead to heartburn or indigestion while chronic worry and/or resentment makes you more susceptible to high blood pressure. However, do not suppress your feelings, even though some may appear irrational to you. Doing so also leads to higher acid levels in your body. Feel the feeling, express it through healthy catharsis in a safe environment if you feel the need to (e.g. screaming into a pillow) – and let it go. Yes, the key here is to let go. Do not dwell on negative feelings.

3. **Meditate daily** – Make meditation a habit. In the long term, meditation brings you peace of mind and makes you more able to cope with stress. It need not be a complex meditation – stillness and emptiness of mind is the key. Sit in a comfortable position and breathe slowly, deeply. Focus on each part of your body and feel it release its tension. After you feel

sufficiently relaxed, you can silently repeat a simple word with no particular emotional attachment for you – for example, you can say "tree." Or, you can actually say a letter, like *a*. Repeat this word or letter in your mind for about one minute. Then sit still and let thoughts come to your mind. Observe your thoughts as if you were apart from them, as though they were another person's thoughts. This is so that you do not dwell on any thought. Just objectively, naturally, allow any thought to enter your mind then leave.

If you reach a state of emptiness, where you feel you are thinking about *nothing*, congratulations! It may take some time for you to reach this point, though.

4. Take up yoga. Not only is this an excellent stress-buster, it also directly fires up your metabolism. The endocrine system and the thyroid help regulate metabolism. Yoga has many positions which give a healthy twist and compression to your endocrine organs, thereby strengthening them for metabolism.

For relaxation from stress, though, a good yoga position is the corpse pose. As its name instructs, you should lie like a corpse. Release all tension from your body. The corpse pose is actually a good ending to your yoga routine.

5. **Plan ahead** – If the cause of your stress is recurring, plan ahead. After you have identified the cause of your stress, ask yourself if there is any way you can avoid it. For example, one cause of your stress may be the morning rush-hour traffic. To be relaxed while you are on your way to work, you have to leave early. Then you remember you watch television every night, sometimes late into the night. To avoid stress in the morning, you conclude you can decrease your television time and go to sleep earlier the night before.

By the way, if your body is subjected to stress such as long working hours, you should modify your diet while still keeping the principles of the fast metabolism diet. You especially need Vitamin C, as this helps the body cope during stress. Load up on citrus fruits and strawberries.

For vegetables, sweet red pepper is an excellent source of Vitamin C. Other than that, your diet remains the same – load up on complex carbohydrates, particularly fibrous ones and take in protein.

Why sleep is important

Sleep is the time your body fully recovers from your workouts. This is also the time that your muscles grow – yes, they do not grow during your workout but while you are in bed. With little sleep, your muscles grow very little even if you put in much effort in your workouts.

Lack of sleep will also prevent your body from being in top form and will thus also affect your energy for workouts. You might find yourself getting tired easily even after a few sets or reps.

Also, scientific studies show that lack of sleep affects carbohydrate metabolism. Glucose is not metabolized as much, resulting in increased hunger and decreased overall metabolism.

It is important for you to get at least eight hours of sleep every night for the body to fully re-charge for the next day.

Although people's circadian rhythms may differ, the normal circadian rhythm is 10 pm to 6 am. This is the best period for muscles to grow. So sleep early to increase your metabolism!

Fit & Slim Checkpoint:

For some, de-stressing may be the most difficult part of the program to boost metabolism. What if stress has become so much a part of your daily life that making serious changes in your lifestyle is difficult? You can take things slowly. The least you need to do, though, is to find some quiet time to yourself every day. It can be as little as ten minutes. Use those ten minutes to just relax and meditate.

Meditation goes a long way. Even ten minutes every day helps you cope better with stress. Studies show that people who meditate regularly are less stressed and are more able to meet life's demands. If there are times you cannot avoid staying up late, catch up on sleep on the weekend. Don't let your sleep "debt" accumulate. Sleep "debt" leads to poor cognitive function and poor health overall. Your body processes don't function as well as they should – and that includes metabolism. Take time to de-stress. It not only boosts your metabolism but also improves your health in general.

So now you know the entire program. But we are not through just yet!

Fit & Slim for Life

Chapter Five

TO BE FIT & SLIM FOR LIFE:

FIRE UP YOUR METABOLSIM NOW!

You have learned all you need to do - now is the best time to start. In sum, you have learned that metabolism is the process of converting calories into energy for storage or immediate use. You now know that metabolism is an essential body function, working every second of your life – even while you are sleeping. And you now know the overall metabolism formula – basal metabolism + physical activity + the thermic effect of food, as well as what factors influence the rate of your metabolism.

Now you already have the knowledge on how to boost your metabolism:

Exercise smart

- Build muscle through a combination of strength and resistance exercises with weights and without weights.

Use exercises that work the most number of muscle groups possible. (2-3 sets, with 6-8 reps each)

- Increase calorie-burning through interval training with cardiovascular exercise. Alternate high-intensity exercise with moderate-intensity exercise. (30 minutes, with one to four minutes per interval.

- Do the two exercises on alternate days throughout the week. Allot one day for total rest with no exercise.

- Metabolic Chain Workouts are great to save time, elevate the intensity of the workout avoid repetitiveness and boredom and have a bit of fun. But do not ever overdue it!

Eat right

- If less is good for traditional weight loss diets, more is good for the fast metabolism diet.

- Stock up on carbohydrates and protein, as these are the driving forces of metabolism.

- Include calcium and healthy fats in your diet.

- Timing is important.

- Always eat breakfast to kick off your metabolism for the day.

- Eat five to six meals in a day, every two and a half to three hours. Never skip meals.

- Drink at least eight glasses of water a day.

- Take one snack or meal within one hour after your workout for the day.

- Don't forget to fill up with fruit and vegetables

   De-stress

- Re-charge through "sensation therapy" (aromatherapy, massage and music) and imagery. For long-term improvement, meditate daily, take up yoga, and think positively. Do not dwell on negative feelings.

- Plan ahead to avoid stressful situations.

So there you have it. What you now need to do is "excuse-proof" your fast metabolism program to ensure you get the best results. In times when you feel little motivation, go back to the scene I asked you to visualize – yourself, after

going through the program. Though people's bodies differ, you

will most likely notice the results in just three or four weeks –

or even two weeks.

Fit & Slim for Life

Chapter Six

CHOOSING THE HEALTHY LIFESTYLE:

The secrets of staying Fit & Slim for life

Once you have reached your target weight, you'll want to know how to maintain it so you don't put all that hard work to waste! Educating yourself ahead of time will help you when you are at the point where you have attained your weight loss goal. You wouldn't want to ruin the celebration you will want to have, and you of course want to continue on with your newfound healthy lifestyle.

• **Don't skip any meals!** Remember, your body's metabolism will take this as a signal that your body is starving and will begin to store fat for reserves. Make sure you keep up with eating your meals, scheduled out as you have been. Besides, if you skip a meal at one point in the day, it could mean you overeat later on when you are just so hungry.

• **Keep eating a variety of foods.** This will help you to keep getting all the nutrients and vitamins your body needs to stay working properly. It will keep you feeling healthy, energized and protect your body by keeping it healthy. You can include choices from whole grains, fruits, vegetables and lean proteins.

• **Keep up the exercising!** Don't get lazy and slack off on your exercise routine now. You have gained the knowledge of what kind of a workout is right for you, and probably how to change it up every once in a while as well if you had instruction from a personal trainer.

Changing up your routine is a great idea to keep you from getting bored, and to keep your body guessing. As long as you are always combining your cardio, metabolic chains and strength training, you will continue to stay fit and feel strong and healthy, all while protecting yourself further from illnesses coupled with your healthy diet.

• **Adjust your daily caloric intake.** Many people wonder if they should increase their daily caloric intake as they increase exercise and daily activity. It is probably advisable to do so, but do so gradually. Try starting with just 250 calories more a day. After a week, weigh yourself. You'll probably have lost some more weight. If this is the case, add another 250 calories, then weight yourself a week after that. Repeat these steps until you see that your weight has remained the same when you weigh yourself for the week. If you gained a bit, take

Fit & Slim for Life

away some calories, 100 at a time, until your weight evens out and remains the same from week to week.

• **Keep drinking that water!** Don't forget to have at least eight glasses of water a day to keep your body working well. Water aides in digestion, increases your energy and helps rid your body of toxins naturally. Plus, you will stay hydrated and healthy.

• **Keep eating frequently.** Eating five to six small meals a day as you have probably already learned to do is a good thing to continue doing, as this keeps your metabolism up, and keeps you feeling satisfied. It is important to continue this as well because you don't want to fall into the trap of increasing your portion sizes again if this was a problem before. You will throw yourself all the way back to square one eventually. In the very least, you will gain a bunch of the weight back you worked so hard to shed.

• **Don't let the junk food back in.** Now that you've developed your healthy habits, why ruin it by going back to your old ways and eating junk food? You have discovered plenty of delicious tastes to satisfy all your cravings with healthy foods. Keep your intake of fruits and vegetables up to several servings a day, preferably 6-8.

The Secrets of Staying Healthy

Everybody wants to live long and healthy lives; nobody wants to count on getting any severe diseases. Although we can't predict or prevent every situation, there are ways to help protect ourselves that can make our lives more full and healthy overall.

• **Prevention and early detection is the first thing you should consider.** Most people dread going for a yearly physical, or even the dentist cleaning every six months, but having good doctors and keeping these appointments in your life will help you to stay healthy because you doctor can detect things that you can't on your own.

Knowing your family history is also important because if there is any history of heart disease or cancers in your family your doctor can keep any eye out for symptoms and do testing on you regularly.

• **Love the people you are with.** Make sure and spend time with the ones who surround you daily such as your spouse, children, other family members, friends and coworkers. Enjoy the time you spend with other people, plus maintain healthy friendships. These relationships are needed to make you feel fulfilled in life.

• **Get eight or more hours of sleep.** Although many people find this one difficult to do because of how busy we can get in our lives, it really is very important to leading a happy and healthy life.

• **Find something you are good at.** All of us have times where we need to be doing something we really enjoy, and most of these are things that we excel at. This is usually something that makes us feel good inside as well, and can even be soothing and stress relieving.

• **Manage your stress – don't ignore it!** Everyone has stressors of some kind, and it is important that we handle our stress so that it does not get out of hand and consume us. When you are riddled with worry and stress it can literally make you sick in many different ways. Daily walks can help clear your head, and make sure that you are not over-filling your agenda for each day or letting other's schedules dictate your day.

• **Find balance in your life.** Don't try to take on too many projects at work or let work consume you. Find a balance so you are still able to enjoy all the other things around you like your hobbies and your friends and family.

Although financial times can be tough, it is still so very important to find time to spend at least with your family, the ones you are working so hard to keep safe and provided for.

The Advantages of Staying Healthy

The benefits of staying healthy are boundless. It doesn't just mean that you are happy with the way you look and can fit into that new outfit. Being healthy has to do with your whole physical, mental and social well-being.

• **Your Physical Health:** Keeping yourself physically healthy can help you all around. Not only can it help you to take part in daily activities such as being able to walk, move and bend, but it allows you to be physically able to take care of your loved ones around you who depend on you.

It can be financially beneficial if you avoid diseases that were preventable and that would be very costly.

• **Your Mental Health:** If you do not have a good mental health, your physical health will also be affected. Many people don't realize just how important their mental health is to their overall well-being. If you allow yourself to be over-stressed or for that stress to rule your life, it can make you sick.

Stress can raise your blood pressure which increases your risk of a heart attack or stroke. You need to deal with your stress in positive ways like through exercise, meditation or therapy. Don't deal with stress by things that can damage your overall health like smoking, drinking or eating unhealthy foods.

• **Disease Prevention:** Making sure you are eating a healthy diet is vital to your overall health and staying healthy. The foods you choose to eat can have a direct impact on your health.

Phytochemicals are important for your health and could prevent things like heart disease, specific types of cancer, diabetes and high blood pressure. They are found only found in certain foods like berries, spinach, olives and kale. Eat a low-fat diet full of lots of fruits and vegetables plus whole grains to help protect your cardiovascular health.

• **Long Life:** Striving to live a healthy lifestyle can be a big factor of you being able to live a long and healthy life. Although you can't prevent all health

problems and some of them are out of your control, a lot of the most significant ones you can help to avoid by living healthy.

With the leading causes of death being chronic diseases such as diabetes, heart disease, stroke and cancer, having lifestyle choices that include controlling the foods you eat, keeping your weight at a healthy level, how much you exercise and how you deal with the stressors in your life can have a huge impact on keeping these diseases at bay.

Living a healthy lifestyle can also improve your mood and give you greater self-esteem and mental focus. You will be stronger, have a higher stamina and you will be able to get a better night's sleep.

Other benefits of a healthy lifestyle include improved digestion and a lower blood pressure. Keeping yourself healthy can also help ease or eliminate back problems and back pain plus improve your posture, enhance coordination and balance, and lower your resting heart rate.

Conclusion

Now that we've learnt how to change your lifestyle and fire your metabolism into action, everybody knows what to do. They read the material, they realize they need to take action and put in the effort but the truth of the matter is people seldom do. Unless you discipline yourself to resist the temptation of eating unhealthy foods and motivate yourself to exercise, relax and eat healthy foods, you will find it difficult to get on the road to a healthy life.

No amount of reading or saying "*Yes, I can do it*" will help you unless you take that first step. It takes a strong commitment to get on track and it takes an equally strong commitment to keep at it. Most people give up after a short time because they're not satisfied with their results. If you can commit and keep yourself motivated and continue to aspire to eat well and train well, you will achieve your goal. No matter what the goal is, be it to lose weight or increase your endurance or become a better athlete in a specific sport, you just need to go out there and make the effort and do the work required.

Over the course of time, not only will you mentally adjust to your training regiment but you will develop a great amount of discipline and self-confidence and you will naturally maintain a positive attitude which means easily being able to resist any kind of temptation. Everybody needs to start from somewhere. Setting your goals little by little as opposed to attempting to go all-out and trying to sweat out 10 pounds on the treadmill in the course of a week will do more harm than good. Starting the process slowly is the key, which means going for a brisk walk to help your body get use to moving before the more rigorous runs you plan to do in the later weeks.

One mistake people make when starting out is going all out which leads to injury and soon they decide that training is just too painful and taxing. As before, set a schedule and if necessary, consult with a personal trainer about what might be good for you if you feel uncomfortable coming up with a schedule. Although you do not need to make the process so difficult. If your desire is to lose weight, all you really require is a small daily window allotted to your exercise and keeping an eye on what you put in your body.

Simply be confident and work towards your goals. Be positive and you will get the results you want.

Fit & Slim for Life

Recipe Book

Because healthy eating isn't a diet,

It's a lifestyle.

Some ideas on how you can use vegetables, herbs, lean protein, nuts and fruits to enjoy healthy, low calorie mains, salads, vegetarian plates and even deserts (29).

Let's get cooking!

Lamb Rack with Cauliflower Mash

Ingredients

- Lamb rack
- Salt and pepper fresh rosemary 2 cloves of garlic, minced
- 1/2 Cauliflower head
- Olive oil

As easy as cooking:

1. Rub salt, pepper, rosemary and 1 clove of garlic onto the lamb rack.
2. Bake at 180C for 20 minutes, or until cooked to your liking.

3. While it is cooking, steam the cauliflower until soft

4. Blend the soften cauliflower in the food processor with remaining garlic, olive oil and more salt and pepper.

5. Enjoy with a large green salad.

Roast Lamb

Ingredients

- 2kg Lamb leg, bone in
- Olive oil
- Rosemary
- Lots of garlic cloves sliced
- Salt and pepper
- Oven pre-heated at 220C

As easy as cooking:

1. Slice small holes in the flesh of the lamb leg and push the rosemary and the sliced garlic in. Rub olive oil and sprinkle salt and pepper over.
2. Place lamb leg in large pot with lid.
3. Place in the oven.
4. Bake at 220C for 1 hour, then turn the oven down to 80C and continue until cooked to your liking.
5. The meat should be tender and falling off the bone.

Lamb & Egg Stack with Avocado & Tomatoes

Ingredients

- 500g Lamb mince, it can also be pork, veal, beef or any lean (less than 4% fat) meat
- 1 Onion, finely chopped
- 2 Cloves of garlic, minced
- Cumin, cinnamon and paprika to taste
- 4 Eggs
- 2 Tomatoes, sliced
- 1 Avocado, sliced
- Salt and pepper
- Coconut oil to fry

As easy as cooking:

1. Mix together the mince, onion, garlic and spices and roll into discs.
2. Fry in an oiled pan until cooked through.
3. Remove from the pan and fry the eggs.
4. Assemble by stacking first the lamb patties, then the egg, then tomato and finally the avocado.

Chicken Patties with Guacamole & Salsa

Ingredients

- 500g Chicken mince
- 1 Avocado
- 1/2 red or yellow pepper, finely diced
- 2 Tomatoes, diced
- 8 Mushrooms, finely diced
- 1/4 Red onion, finely diced
- Juice of 1⁄2 a lemon
- 1 Cloves of garlic, minced
- Salt and pepper
- Chilli flakes (optional, but it's worth trying!)
- Cumin to taste
- Coconut oil to fry

For the Salsa

- Paprika to taste
- Chilli flakes to taste
- 1 Small onion, finely diced
- 8 tomatoes
- Juice of ½ lemon
- Zest of 1 lemon
- 1 Clove of garlic, minced
- Pepper and salt to taste

As easy as cooking:

1. Mix together the chicken mince, pepper, mushrooms, onion, garlic, salt, pepper, cumin and paprika and roll them into small, flat discs.
2. Fry in an oiled pan until cooked through.
3. Mix avocado, 2 tomatoes, onion, lemon and chilli together with a fork, until you reach desired guacamole consistency.
4. In a food processor, blend the salsa ingredients and chill before serving
5. Stack the guacamole on top of each disc, top some salsa over and enjoy with a green salad.

Spiced Mince Meat

Ingredients

- 500g beef mince, it can also be pork, veal, chicken, lamb or any lean (less than 4% fat) meat
- 1 Large onion, diced
- 200g Green beans, diced
- Cumin
- Ginger
- Garlic Salt and pepper
- Ground coriander to taste

As easy as cooking:

1. Fry the onion and beans in an oiled pan, add mince and spices and break up with your spatula to avoid clumps.
2. When the mixture is cooked through, serve in a bowl with red pepper strips as dippers

Mexican Ground Turkey Mix for Tacos, Fajitas, Salads and more

Ingredients

- 4 cloves of garlic
- 500g organic ground turkey
- 1 tsp cumin
- Black pepper to taste
- ½ Red onion chopped
- Garlic salt
- Paprika to taste
- ½ fresh chilli or chilli powder
- ½ tsp oregano
- ½ cup water
- Coconut oil to sauté
- Hot sauce to taste
-

As easy as cooking:

1. Heat pan over medium high heat.

Fit & Slim for Life

2. Add garlic and sauté until soft and add the turkey
3. Using spoon break turkey into small pieces and cook for 3-4 minutes or until meat starts to become brown.
4. Mix all spices in small bowl and add to turkey mixture and stir to combine.
5. Add water and bring to a simmer.
6. Cook for further 5 minutes

Chicken & Olives

Ingredients

- 2 Chicken breasts
- 1 Onion, diced
- Salt & pepper
- 1 Jar of olives
- 1500ml Jar of basil and tomato pasta sauce, look for a sugar free one or give it a go making your own.
- Coconut oil to cook
- Parmesan cheese to serve
-

As easy as cooking:

1. Brown the chicken in an oiled pan with onion, salt and pepper.
2. Add the pasta sauce and olives, tip into a baking dish
3. Bake at 180C for 30 minutes

Fit & Slim for Life

4. Serve with some parmesan cheese sprinkles.

Mediterranean Chicken Stack

Ingredients

- 4 Chicken thighs or breast, hammered flat
- Salt and pepper
- 1 Clove of garlic, finely chopped
- Baby spinach
- 8 Sundried tomatoes
- Olives
- Fresh basil
- Coconut oil to fry

As easy as cooking:

1. Fry the chicken in an oiled pan with salt, pepper and garlic until cooked through (about 5 minutes per side).
2. 2. Stack the chicken on top of the spinach and top with sundried tomatoes, olives and basil.

Roast Chicken

Ingredients

- Whole chicken

- 3-4 Slices of preserved lemon (lemons marinated in oil and salt for a few weeks if you want to make it yourself)
- Olive oil
- Salt and pepper
- Pre-heated oven at 180C
- Loads of green vegetables to serve with

As easy as cooking:

1. Place chicken in a large pot with a lid.
2. Drizzle with olive oil, lay the lemon slices on top and sprinkle with salt and pepper.
3. Put the lid on and bake at 180C for 1 hour and 20 minutes.
4. Check that the meat is cooked by slicing into the thigh with a knife – if the juices run clear, the meat is cooked. If not, leave it for an extra 10 minutes.
5. Serve with green vegetables. Delicious paired with coleslaw!

Chicken, Chilli, Prawn & Kelp Noodles

Ingredients

- 400g Kelp noodles (from a health, vegetarian or vegan shop)
- 4 Tbsp coconut oil

- 2 Chicken breasts, thinly sliced
- 16 Raw peeled prawns, heads removed
- 150g Choy sum or Bok Choy or any Chinese greens you like, cut into matchsticks if you don't like them, try cabbage instead.
- 2 Tbsp tamari
- 2 Tbsp rice wine vinegar
- 1 Tbsp honey
- 1 tsp Chilli paste
- 1 Handful beansprouts
- 1/2 Cup fresh coriander leaves
- 3 Tbsp crispy shallots
- ½ lemon

As easy as cooking:

1. Prepare the kelp noodles as per the package and plate.
2. Heat coconut oil in a wok until smoking.
3. Add the sliced chicken and cook for 2-3 minutes or until nicely colored.
4. Add the prawns and Choy sum matchsticks and cook for 2 more minutes, add sauces, then the chilli paste.
5. Toss in the beansprouts.
6. Fold in the coriander, serve immediately on kelp noodles, and garnish with crispy shallots and a squeeze of lemon.

Roast Pork with Baked Vegetables

Ingredients

- 1 Pork loin (approximately 2kg, bone in)
- 1/2 Cauliflower, chopped
- Salt and pepper
- 1/2 Broccoli, chopped
- 4 carrots
- A bunch of asparagus
- Minced garlic
- 1 Onion, chopped
- Paprika
- 2 Cloves of garlic, finely diced
- Cumin
- 2 Slices of preserved lemons
- Oregano
- Olive oil
- 2 Cups of water
- Oven pre-heated at 200C

As easy as cooking:

1. Place the pork skin side up in a large roasting pan with a lid. Rub the salt, pepper, garlic, spices and olive oil

into the fat, add 2 cups of water to the pan, cover and put in the oven at 200C for 30 minutes.

2. Turn the oven down to 140C and continue cooking for another 5 hours at least.

3. Check the meat after this; it should be tender and falling off the bone. You may need to leave it for another couple of hours, just keep checking for when the bone slides out easily.

4. Cover and leave to rest while vegetables cook.

5. Place cauliflower, carrots, broccoli and onion on a baking tray, sprinkle with garlic, lemon and oil and bake at 200C for 30-40 minutes until cooked through.

6. Just before serving, snap the hard ends off and steam the asparagus for 3 to 4 minutes.

7. Enjoy an amazing family dinner!

Mince Lettuce Cups

Ingredients

- 1kg Pork/chicken/beef mince or cooked and flaked white fish meat or crab meat
- 1 Large lettuce, leaves torn off
- Tamari soy sauce
- Tomatoes, sliced

- Fish sauce
- Coconut oil to fry
- 1 Large white onion, diced
- 2 Cloves of garlic, crushed or sliced thinly
- Chilli flakes/fresh chilli, sliced thinly
- Salt and pepper
- Olive oil and a big squeeze of lemon to serve
- Avocado (optional)

As easy as cooking:

1. Combine mince, tamari soy sauce, fish sauce, onion, garlic, chilli, salt and pepper together.
2. Heat some coconut oil in a large frying pan, add the mince mixture and fry until the meat is cooked all the way through. Skip this step is you are using already cooked and flaked white fish meat or crab.
3. Serve with the lettuce leaves by spooning mixture and tomatoes, squeeze lemon and drizzle olive oil into the lettuce cups.
4. Now, eat it with your hands, sort of like lettuce tacos, and don't forget the avocado!

Chilli with sweet potato mash

Ingredients

- 500g Mince
- 1 Onion, chopped
- 2 Cloves of garlic
- Green beans, diced
- Big pepper, diced
- 2 Tins tomatoes
- Cinnamon
- Chilli flakes
- Cumin
- Paprika
- Salt and pepper
- Coconut oil to fry
- Large sweet potato, peeled
- Drop of milk and a bit of real butter

As easy as cooking:

1. Fry the vegetables in coconut oil in a large heavy saucepan.
2. Add the mince, tomatoes and spices, and simmer for 20 minutes.
3. Boil the sweet potato until soft, mash with a bit of milk, butter and a pinch of salt

4. Serve for a warming supper!

Spiced Beef Short Ribs

Ingredients

- 1.2 - 1.4kg Beef short ribs
- 2 Cups vegetable stock, hot
- 1 Onion, chopped
- 1 Carrot, chopped
- 1 Leek, white part only, thinly sliced
- 25g Coconut oil, softened
- 1 Tbsp almond/coconut flour
- 4 Cloves of garlic, peeled
- 1 Tbsp bittersweet smoked paprika
- 1/2 Tbsp hot smoked paprika (or use all bittersweet)
- 1/2 Tbsp cumin seeds, toasted, crushed
- 1/2 Tbsp honey
- 1/2 tsp Salt
- Loads of green-leaf vegetables

As easy as cooking:

1. Combine the paprika, cumin, honey and salt in a small bowl and set aside.
2. Preheat a slow cooker for 20 minutes then put in the onion, carrot, leek and whole garlic cloves.

3. Using your hands, rub the paprika mix all over the beef short ribs then put them on top of the vegetables. Then pour in the hot stock, cover and cook on Low for 7-8 hours.
4. Remove the short ribs form the slow cooker and keep warm. Strain the cooking juices, pushing down on the vegetables, into a wide saucepan or frying pan and bring to the boil.
5. Mix the oil and flour to a paste then whisk this paste into the cooking juices, to make a thin sauce.
6. When ready to serve, cut the short ribs between each bone and serve with the sauce
7. Just before serving, steam the green-leaf vegetables for 2 or 3 minutes and serve.

Surf & Turf

- Beef tenderloin or eye fillet per person
- 6 Prawns per person
- Coconut aioli
- Green salad

As easy as cooking:

1. Fry eye fillet for 3 minutes each side.
2. Add the prawns for the final few minutes of cooking.

3. Serve with a green salad or asparagus and drizzle over the coconut aioli.

Prawns & Cabbage

Ingredients

- 500g Raw prawn meat
- 1 Onion, diced
- 2 Cloves of garlic, crushed
- 1/2 Head of cabbage
- 1/2 Can of coconut milk
- Juice of 1 lemon
- Salt and pepper to taste

As easy as cooking:

1. Fry the onion and garlic in an oiled pan.
2. Add the cabbage, let it soften, and then add the prawns.
3. Pour over the coconut milk, lemon juice, salt and pepper and let it simmer for 5 minutes.
4. Delicious served with a large green salad!

Poached Prawns

Ingredients

- Raw prawn meat
- Fresh orange juice
- Coconut milk
- Garlic, crushed
- Salt and pepper

As easy as cooking:

1. Mix everything together and marinate for 1 hour.
2. Remove prawns from liquid and set aside.
3. Heat liquid in a pot, and add prawns and poach until cooked through.
4. Serve with Couscous!

Vegetable Frittata

Ingredients

- 12 Eggs
- 1 Yellow or red pepper, sliced thinly
- 1 Onion, sliced thinly
- 3 Tomatoes, diced
- 2 Cloves of garlic, diced or crushed
- 2 Zucchinis, sliced thinly
- Coconut oil for fraying
- Fresh chilli (optional)
- Salt and pepper

As easy as cooking:

1. Whisk eggs. Set aside.
2. In a large oven-proof saucepan, fry the vegetables in a little coconut oil until tender.
3. Remove from the heat, add the egg mix and salt and pepper to taste.
4. Bake in the oven for 20 minutes or until eggs are cooked through.
5. Serve with a large green salad.

Cabbage with Sesame & Ginger

Ingredients

- 1 Cabbage, shredded
- 1 Tbsp sesame oil
- 1 Tbsp fresh root ginger, grated
- 1 Clove of garlic, crushed
- Salt and pepper

As easy as cooking:

1. Heat 1 inch of water in a saucepan, add the cabbage, cover with a lid and cook for about 5 minutes, or until the cabbage is tender. Drain.
2. Add the sesame oil, ginger and garlic and stir well.
3. Season with salt and pepper and serve immediately.

Fit & Slim for Life

Naked Huevos Rancheros

- 2 Eggs
- 1 yellow or red pepper, sliced
- 1⁄4 Red onion, sliced
- 1 Avocado, sliced
- 1 Large tomato, sliced
- Salsa, to taste
- Fresh coriander, to taste
- Salt and pepper

As easy as cooking:

1. Whisk eggs and fry in an oiled pan. This is your tortilla.
2. Place the veggies, salsa and coriander on cooked egg and wrap around.
3. Enjoy!

Kale Salad

Ingredients

- 1 Bag of kale, chopped finely
- 10 Mushrooms, sliced
- 2 Cloves of garlic, minced
- 1⁄2 Onion, sliced very finely

- Balsamic vinegar
- Olive oil
- Salt and pepper

As easy as cooking:

1. Mix kale, mushrooms, garlic and onion together.
2. Dress salad with olive oil, balsamic vinegar, salt and pepper.

Coleslaw

Ingredients

- Grated carrot
- Red cabbage, sliced thinly
- 1 Onion, sliced thinly
- Organic, high quality Mayonnaise
- Lemon Juice

As easy as cooking:

1. Mix everything together in a big bowl.
2. Enjoy!

Carrots with Nutty Dressing

Ingredients

Fit & Slim for Life

- 3 Tbsp organic nut butter (unsweetened peanut or almond or any other organic blend)
- 2 tsp Tumeric
- 3 Cloves of garlic, minced
- 1/2 Cup olive oil
- 3 Carrots, grated

As easy as cooking:

1. Combine nut butter, turmeric, garlic and enough olive oil until good dressing consistency and smooth.
2. Mix into the carrots.
3. Enjoy!

Broccoli & Green Bean Salad

Ingredients

- Broccoli
- Green beans
- Avocado
- Chilli
- Lemon juice Balsamic vinegar
- Salt and pepper

As easy as cooking:

1. Steam broccoli florets and green beans until slightly tender, remove from pot and let cool.
2. Toss with avocado, chilli, lemon juice, salt and pepper and a dash of balsamic vinegar.

Coconut Aioli

Ingredients

- 250g Organic unsweetened coconut yoghurt
- 1 Tbsp garlic, crushed
- 1 tsp Sea salt
- Juice of 1 lemon
- Pepper

As easy as cooking:

1. Combine all the ingredients and mix well.
2. Drizzle over salads, chicken or fish, or serve with Crudités

Raspberry Cooler Drink (Low Carb) Makes 3 cups

Ingredients

- 1 cup raspberries, frozen or fresh
- 1 ½ cups water

- ¼ cup heavy cream
- ½ tsp vanilla extract
- 1-2 cups ice cubes (to desired thickness)
- Liquid stevia, organic honey or organic agave syrup to desired sweetness

As easy as cooking:

1. Combine raspberries, water, cream and vanilla in a blender or food processor until smooth
2. Add ice cubes, one at a time until desired consistency
3. Add liquid stevia, honey or syrup to taste and garnish with mint leafs.

Coconut Bars

Ingredients

- 3 eggs
- 1 cup coconut milk
- ⅓ cup coconut oil
- ⅓ cup coconut nectar
- 1 tablespoon vanilla
- ⅛ teaspoon liquid stevia, if you can find vanilla crème stevia drops
- ½ cup almond flour
- 1 tablespoon coconut flour

- 1 ½ cups unsweetened shredded coconut
- ¼ teaspoon sea salt

As easy as cooking:

1. Mix eggs, coconut milk, oil, nectar, vanilla and stevia in a food processor
2. Add in almond flour, coconut flour, shredded coconut and salt
3. Transfer ingredients into an 8x8 inch baking dish, layered with baking paper
4. Bake at 350C for 30 minutes
5. Cool for hour
6. Cut into bars and place in refrigerator. Serve when chilled

Coconut Macaroons

Ingredients

- 1 package unsweetened coconut flour
- 4-5 egg whites
- 1-2 TB liquid sweetener (coconut nectar, stevia or honey)
- 2 tsp vanilla
- 8-10 oz dark chocolate
- Preheat oven to 400.

Fit & Slim for Life

As easy as cooking:

1. Mix all ingredients except chocolate together.
2. Form golf ball sized balls and place on lightly greased baking sheet
3. Bake until golden brown, roughly 15 minutes while macaroons are baking, melt chocolate on low heat on stove.
4. Take macaroons out of oven; allow cooling for 10 minutes
5. Roll macaroons in the chocolate for a lovely decoration.

Good luck and good health for all.

Fit & Slim for Life

DISCLAIMER AND LEGAL NOTICES

The information presented within this book solely and fully represents the views of the author as of the date of publication. Any slight to, or potential misrepresentation of, any peoples or companies is entirely unintentional. As a result of changing information, conditions or contexts, this author reserves the right to alter content or option with impunity.

This e-book does not in any way substitute for medical or psychological/psychiatric advice or recommendation. You should always consult with your doctor or other qualified professional regarding any known or suspected medical or mental condition or illness, as well as before engaging in any form of exercise or making any change to your dietary practices. You should always consult with a doctor prior to beginning any new medical regimen, including changing or introducing medications, supplements, or other therapeutic procedures. This e-book does not substitute for professional medical advice or recommendation, and as such the author and the author's re sellers and affiliates cannot assume responsibility for any outcome or effect on the reader's well-being or health in any way whatsoever. You should always consult with a professional if you are or think you may be experiencing any sort of health condition or disorder or disease.

This e-book is for informational purposes only and the author does not accept any responsibility for any sort liability, including injury, stress, strain, debility or financial loss, resulting from the use of this information.

This information is not presented by a medical or psychological practitioner and is for educational and informational purposes only. The content is not intended to be a substitute for professional medical advice, diagnosis, or treatment. Always seek the advice of your physician or other qualified health care provider with any questions you may have regarding a medical condition. Never disregard professional medical advice or delay in seeking it because of something you have read or heard.

While every attempt has been made to verify the information contained herein, the author and the author's re-sellers and affiliates cannot assume any responsibility for errors, inaccuracies, or omissions.

References

Fit & Slim for Life

Bosello, O., & Zamboni, M. (2000). Visceral obesity and metabolic syndrome. *Obesity reviews,1*(1)(2), 47-56.

Food and Nutrition Board, Institute of Medicine. Dietary Reference Intakes for Energy, Carbohydrate, Fiber, Fat, Fatty Acids, Cholesterol, Protein, and Amino Acids. Washington, DC: National Academy Press, 2002.(3)

Volek, J. S., Sharman, M. J., Love, D. M., Avery, N. G., Scheett, T. P., & Kraemer, W. J. (2002). Body composition and hormonal responses to a carbohydrate-restricted diet. *Metabolism, 51*(7), 864-870. (4) (5)

Dolezal BA, Potteiger JA. Concurrent resistance and endurance training influence basal metabolic rate in nondieting individuals. Journal of Applied Physiology. 1998;85(2):695-700 (6)

Hensrud D. Slow metabolism: Is it to blame for weight gain? Rochester, MN: Mayo Foundation for Medical Education and Research (MFMER); [updated 2011 Aug 23; cited 2013 June 6]. Available from:
http://www.mayoclinic.com . (7)

What is metabolism? Tarzana, CA: Metabolic Institute of America (MIA); [cited 2013 June 6]. Available from:http://www.themetaboliccenter.com. (8)

Scott Plisk S. Anaerobic Metabolic Conditioning: A brief Review of Theory, Strategy and Practical Application. Journal of Applied Sport Science Research 1991, Volume5, Number 1 pp. 24-34. Available from:
http://www.unm.edu/~lkravitz/Sports%20Physiology/Plisk.pdf
(9)

Robert Reames, Trainer. Makeover your Metabolism, Jenson Books Inc. Available from http://www.fitnessmagazine.com/workout/lose-weight/make-over-your-metabolism-robert-reames-secrets-to-fat-burning-success/ (10) (11) (15)

Eur J Appl Physion Occup Shysiol 1999. Miller AE, MacDougall JD, Tarnopolsky MA, Sale DG, Gender Differences in strength and muscle fibre characteristics. Available from
http://www.ncbi.nlm.nih.gov/pubmed/8477683 (12) (13)

TANAKA, H. et al. (2001) Age-predicted maximal heart rate revisited. *Journal of the American College of Cardiology, 37* (1), p. 153-156 (16) Available from
http://content.onlinejacc.org/article.aspx?articleid=1126908&resultClick=3#tab1 (16)

Med Sci Sports Exerc. 2009 Mar;41(3):687-708. doi: 10.1249/MSS.0b013e3181915670. American College of Sport Medicine position stand. Progression models in resistance training for healthy adults. Available from http://www.ncbi.nlm.nih.gov/pubmed/19204579 (14) (17)

Talanian, Jason L., et al. "Two weeks of high-intensity aerobic interval training increases the capacity for fat oxidation during exercise in women." *Journal of applied physiology* 102.4 (2007): 1439-1447. Available from http://www.ncbi.nlm.nih.gov/pubmed/17170203 (18)

J Laforgia, RT Withers & CJ George. Journal of Sports Sciences Volume 24, Issue 12, 2006. Original Articles: Effects of exercise intensity and duration on the excess post-exercise oxygen consumption. Pages 1247 – 126. Available from http://www.tandfonline.com/doi/abs/10.1080/02640410600552064 (19)

Wayne t, Phillips PhD, FACSM, Tannah E. Broman Ms, Lee N, Burkett Phd & Pamela D Swann PhD, FACSM. Activities, Adaptation & Aging Volume 27, Issue 3-4, 2003. Original Articles: Single Set Strength Training Increases Strength, Endurance and Functional Fitness in Community Living Older Adults. Available from http://www.tandfonline.com/doi/abs/10.1300/J016v27n03_01 (20)

Monica Dinu Msc, Rosanna Abbate MD, Gian Franco Gensini,MD, Alessandro CAsini MD & Francesco Sofi MD, PhD 2006. Critical Reviews in Food Science and Nutrition. Original Articles: Vegetarian, vegan diets and multiple health outcomes: a systematic review with meta-analysis of observational studies. Available from http://www.tandfonline.com/doi/full/10.1080/10408398.2016.1138447 (21)

Jessica Elizabeth De La Torre Torres, Fatma Gassara, Anne Patricia Kouassi, Satinder Kaur Brar & Khaled Belkacemi. Critical Reviews in Food Science and Nutrition 2015. Original Articles: Spice Use in Food: Properties and Benefits. Available from http://www.tandfonline.com/doi/full/10.1080/10408398.2013.858235 (22)

KJ Ellis. Journal of the American College of Nutrition, Volume 13, Issue 3, 1994. Editorial Body Composition, obesity and weight loss. Pages 220-2201. Available from

http://www.tandfonline.com/doi/abs/10.1080/07315724.1994.1
0718399 (23)

KL Tamashiro, RR Sakai, CA Shivelry, IN Karatsoreo & LP Ragan. The
International Journal on the Biology of Stress. Chronic Stress, Metabolism
and Metabolic Syndrome. Pages 468 – 474. Available from
http://www.tandfonline.com/doi/full/10.3109/10253890.2011.6
06341 (24)

AB Crujeiras, A Diasz-Lagares, MC Carreira, M Amil & FF Casanueva. Free
Radical Research Volume 47, Issue 4, 2013. Oxidative stress associated to
dysfunctional adipose tissue: a potential link between obesity, type 2
diabetes mellitus and breast cancer. Available from
http://www.tandfonline.com/doi/full/10.3109/10715762.2013.7
72604 (25)

An Pelt RE et al. Regular exercise and the age -related decline in resting
metabolic rate in women. J Clin Endocrinol Metab. 1997 Oct;82: 3208-12
(26)

van Pelt, R.E., Dinneno, F.A., Seals, D.R., & Jones, P.P. (2001). Age-related
decline in RMR in physically active men: relation to exercise volume and
energy intake. American Journal of Physiology, E281, 633-639 (27)

Why I love Coconut Oil:
http://www.lifestylebypoliquin.com/Lifestyle/Nutrition/504/_
Why_I_Love_Coconut_Oil.aspx (28)

Assuncao ML et al. Effectos of dietary coconut oil on the bieochemical and
antrhopometric profiles of women presenting abdominal obsity. Lipids. 2009
Jul:44:593-601 (28)

For more recepies (29), visit
http://www.lesmills.com/knowledge/nutrition/21-day-
challenge-recipe-download/